Introduction   5

Allergy: an increasing problem   7

Allergens: the causes of allergy   11

Diagnosing allergy   17

Pathogenesis   22

Therapeutic principles   27

Seasonal allergic rhinitis   36

Perennial rhinitis: allergic and non-allergic   38

Nasal polyposis: a non-allergic disease   43

Associated diseases   47

Key references   49

Index   52

Introduction

Allergic diseases have been described as a modern epidemic, with over 20% of the total population suffering from allergic rhinitis, asthma or atopic eczema. Of these diseases, allergic rhinitis is the most common. Severely affected patients are treated by specialists in allergy, lung medicine, otorhinolaryngology and dermatology. The majority of patients, however, are dealt with by generalists or by specialists in other fields. It is for them that this short and practically oriented text on allergic rhinitis has been written.

CHAPTER 1
Allergy: an increasing problem

Atopic diseases

The term 'atopy' refers to a genetic predisposition to produce IgE in response to minute amounts of environmental protein allergens. Non-atopic individuals can produce IgE, but normally do so only transiently. In atopics, the production continues and leads to various atopic disorders, such as:

- atopic dermatitis or eczema
- asthma
- allergic rhinitis.

A highly atopic patient is affected early in life, developing atopic dermatitis soon after birth; asthma and allergic rhinitis develop subsequently. On the other hand, a person who becomes pollen allergic in adolescence has a low degree of atopy and is unlikely to be troubled by asthma and eczema. Fortunately, the latter scenario is more common.

Epidemiology. Twenty to thirty per cent of the population of the industrialized world has a positive skin-prick test for allergens, and 15–20% will develop an atopic disease. The prevalence of atopic diseases is highest during the teenage years. Skin-prick tests remain positive even after symptoms have disappeared.

Allergic rhinitis, atopic dermatitis and asthma have increased in prevalence in western and westernized countries in the past 30–40 years (Figures 1.1 and 1.2). The reason for this is unknown, but a switch from protective IgG-type immune reactions (mediated by T-helper 1 cells; Th1 cells) to allergic IgE-type ones (T-helper 2 cells; Th2 cells) in response to decreased infection in early years has been postulated. These T-helper lymphocyte subsets are characterized by their cytokine profile; Th1 synthesize interleukin-2 (IL-2) and interferon-γ, while Th2 cells produce IL-4, IL-5 and IL-13. The Th1 and Th2 systems are mutually suppressive. It is in accordance with this hypothesis that seasonal allergic rhinitis is more common in first-born children and in higher social classes, in whom infectious contacts are less frequent.

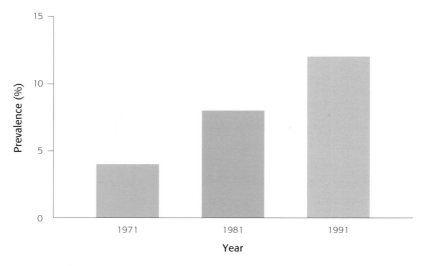

Figure 1.1 The increasing prevalence of allergic rhinitis in young Swedish men. Reproduced with permission from Åberg N. *Clin Exp Allergy* 1989;19:59–63.

Other possibly important factors are the decrease in breastfeeding and increased exposure to house-dust mites in poorly ventilated homes with high humidity. Although it is an unpleasant conclusion to draw, we do not fully understand the reasons for the considerable increase in the prevalence of allergic rhinitis that has occurred over recent decades.

Development. This depends on:
- genetic make up
- allergen exposure
- exposure to 'adjuvants' that facilitate allergic sensitization (possibly).

Genetic factors. With one atopic parent, the risk of atopy in the child is doubled, with maternal influence being greater than paternal. If both parents are atopic, the risk is quadrupled. Several genes are involved and children probably inherit a predisposition for atopic disease in general, specific organ involvement and disease severity. Thus a child with one parent with hay fever is likely to be less severely affected than one whose parents have severe eczema and asthma.

Environmental exposure. A low concordance rate for atopy among monozygotic twins shows that genetic inheritance is not the sole arbiter of

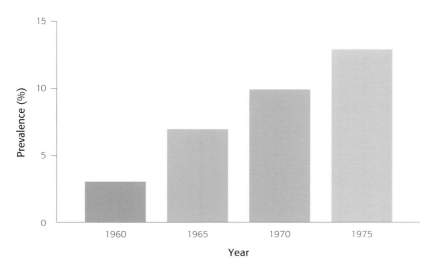

Figure 1.2 The increasing prevalence of atopic dermatitis (eczema) in Danish children according to year of birth. Reproduced with permission from Larsen FS, Hanifin JM. *Acta Derm Venereol Suppl (Stockh)* 1992;176:7–12.

the atopic state. Exposure to aero-allergens is the primary cause of the development of childhood asthma and rhinitis, with mite exposure increasing the risk by 5–10 fold. Similarly, cat and dog dander, cockroach and mould allergens can increase the prevalence of allergic rhinitis and asthma. This has the therapeutic implication that some cases of asthma and allergic rhinitis can be prevented in susceptible infants by allergen avoidance during the early years.

Birth immediately before a pollen season leads to a slightly increased risk of pollen allergy. This is probably because allergen exposure occurs at a time when the immune system is immature and vulnerable.

Both indoor pollution (parental smoking, gas heating) and outdoor pollution (diesel exhaust particles, nitrogen dioxide) can provoke wheezing in sensitized individuals. The role of pollution in allergic sensitization remains in dispute. Table 1.1 illustrates that a higher standard of living is a more important factor than air pollution.

There is convincing evidence that the prevalence of atopic disease increases when people move to industrialized countries from native environments. A study has demonstrated that atopic diseases are more common in affluent

TABLE 1.1

Prevalence of allergic rhinitis among 9- to 11-year-old children in two German cities with different levels of air pollution*

	Leipzig	Munich
Sulphur dioxide ($\mu g/m^3$)	204	11
Particulate matters ($\mu g/m^3$)	134	51
Hay fever (%)	2.4	8.6

*Reproduced from von Mutius *et al. BMJ* 1992;305:1395–9

Munich (former West Germany) than in Leipzig (former East Germany), despite the greater industrial pollution in the latter (Table 1.1).

Non-atopic disease

Some individuals with asthma, rhinitis or nasal polyps are skin-prick test negative yet, as in atopic allergy, Th2-cell-driven and eosinophil-dominated inflammatory reactions are the underlying immunological and pathological features. The aetiology of these disorders is unknown. An example of a non-allergic, allergy-like disorder is intolerance of acetylsalicylic acid (aspirin). These individuals start with rhinitis, progress to nasal polyposis and frequently develop late-onset asthma. Inadvertent ingestion of aspirin can cause severe rhinorrhoea and asthma, which can be life-threatening. Other individuals react with urticaria, angio-oedema and anaphylaxis. It is not an allergic manifestation as the skin-prick test for aspirin is negative and the reaction extends to other non-steroidal anti-inflammatory drugs that are chemically different.

Aspirin intolerance usually develops in middle-aged people – it is extremely rare during childhood. Diagnosis is based on history and, in selected cases, oral provocation testing. Management consists of strict, lifelong avoidance.

CHAPTER 2
Allergens: the causes of allergy

Characteristics

Those antigens that elicit an IgE response are termed 'allergens'. Allergenic extracts (e.g. from house-dust mites) contain several different molecules. Some of these evoke a response in many patients and are termed 'major' allergens. The remainder (minor allergens) affects only a small proportion of patients.

Each allergen molecule comprises a number of antigenic determinants – epitopes. These are small polypeptides, recognized by the immune system as being 'non-self'. Patients vary in their response to different allergen molecules and to different epitopes of the same allergen molecule. As there may be amino-acid sequence similarities between different allergens, cross-reactivity (partial immunological identity) can occur (e.g. between birch pollen and hazelnut).

Measurement

Environmental allergens can be quantified; for example, pollens can be sampled in a pollen trap, and mite and animal allergens can be assessed immunochemically from vacuum-cleaner dust. Mould spores can be collected on culture plates and counted. At present, such measures are largely used in epidemiological investigations and research, but they are also useful clinically.

Pollen

Pollen grains are the gametes of plants and need to be transferred from one plant to another (Figure 2.1). Insect-pollinated plants usually have bright flowers and produce small numbers of pollens; these rarely cause allergy. Wind-pollinated plants release large quantities of small pollen grains and are the major cause of allergy. Since the majority of pollen grains (20–30 µm in size) are trapped in the nose, rhinitis is the usual result. However, pollen allergens released in dew and raindrops have the potential to reach the bronchi as dust and to cause asthma.

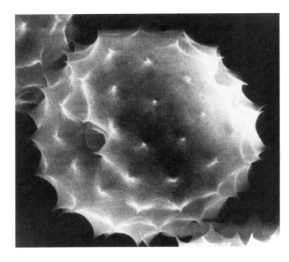

Figure 2.1 A pollen grain as seen with the scanning electron microscope. Pollens are the most important cause of hay fever.

Grass pollen is the most common cause of pollinosis worldwide, affecting over 95% of seasonal allergic rhinitis patients in the UK. Grasses pollinate in the summer (Figure 2.2). As grass species cross-react extensively, the number of extracts needed for diagnosis and treatment is limited. Bermuda grass, however, is a separate entity.

Pollen is released early in the morning, rises high into the atmosphere and descends in the evening as the air cools. The pollen season travels northward at about 5° longitude per week, thus it may be possible to plan a pollen avoidance holiday.

Trees pollinate mainly in the spring; the season is short. In northern Europe, Asia and North America, birch pollen is the main cause of allergy. It is cross-reactive with hazel pollen and nut, and some patients suffer 'birch/apple syndrome', whereby fresh apples and certain vegetables and soft fruit cause oral allergy symptoms.

In Mediterranean areas, the olive tree is the major cause of pollen allergy.

Weeds. Ragweed is a major cause of seasonal allergic rhinitis in North America. Its season runs between mid-August and September. Ragweed plants are extensive in grain fields and ragweed allergy is therefore most prevalent in the midwest region of the USA. The season is later in more southerly areas, in contrast to the grass pollen season.

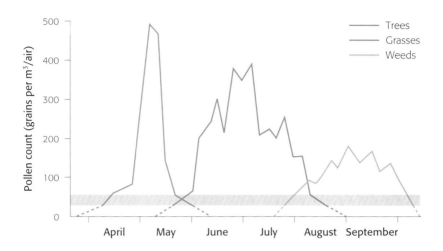

Figure 2.2 The three pollen seasons in the northern hemisphere. Typical pollen counts for a tree season in the spring, grass in summer and weed in early autumn. Most patients develop symptoms when the pollen count reaches 25–50 grains/m^3 of air.

In Europe, mugwort and parietaria are important weed allergen sources. The latter is a perennial weed found in the Mediterranean basin.

Moulds

Moulds or microfungi are microscopic organisms that produce very large numbers of small spores (2–5 µm). These spores can reach the lower airways and therefore tend to cause asthma rather than allergic rhinitis.

Moulds need conditions of high relative humidity in order to grow. They are, therefore, prevalent in temperate climates during the late summer, but are present in the tropics in large quantities all year. In buildings with damp indoor areas moulds can be a problem, particularly if disseminated via the air-conditioning system. The main pathogens are *Cladosporium*, *Alternaria*, *Aspergillus*, *Penicillium* and *Mucor*.

House-dust mites

These creatures, which are just too small to be seen with the naked eye, are the most common indoor source of allergen (Figure 2.3). *Dermatophagoides*

13

pteronyssinus and *Dermatophagoides farinae*, which have strong cross-reactivity, are the most significant species.

Occurrence. Mites require a high relative humidity to survive, as they have no water conservation system. They also breed best at warm temperatures, around 25°C. Ideal conditions exist in mattresses where they have food (human skin scales), warmth and moisture. They also live in carpets, curtains, furniture, pillows, duvets and stuffed toys.

The prevalence of house-dust mites in housing has increased over recent decades, reflecting the increasing numbers of energy-efficient, poorly ventilated, centrally heated and carpeted houses.

Geographical variations. Mites are a worldwide problem; the only areas relatively spared are those deserts with a very dry climate or places at high altitudes (above 3000 m).

Allergens. The major house-dust mite allergens are the digestive enzymes, which are present in their faecal pellets. These are of similar size to pollen grains and are rendered airborne during dusting and cleaning but settle rapidly (within 30 minutes). Highest exposure to mites occurs during sleep.

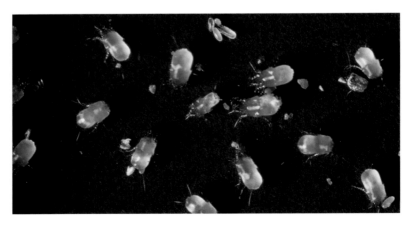

Figure 2.3 House-dust mites seen alive with the stereomicroscope. They are the most important cause of perennial allergic rhinitis. Courtesy of MJ Colloff, Scottish Parasite Diagnostic Laboratory, Stobhill Hospital, Glasgow, UK.

Storage mites

These pests are harboured in stored foods, such as grain in warehouses, granaries, food and farm stores. They are very sensitive to desiccation and are a common cause of allergy in farmers and inhabitants of the tropics. Storage mites do not cross-react with the *Dermatophagoides* species and extracts of storage mites (*Glycophagus*, *Tyrophagus* and *Acarus*) must be included for adequate allergy investigation in some parts of the world.

Cockroaches

In some inner city areas (e.g. Chicago and New York), a high proportion of patients with rhinitis and/or asthma are skin-prick test positive to cockroach extract.

Mammals

Cats and dogs. Over 50% of homes in northern Europe and North America have at least one cat or dog; allergy to these pets is a common cause of symptoms.

In cats, the major allergen is produced in the salivary glands. Dried saliva in the pelt becomes airborne as small sticky allergenic particles which become attached to carpets, furniture and walls. These particles remain in the home for about 6 months after the removal of the cat.

In dogs, the major allergens are from the salivary glands, skin scales and urine. Hair itself is not allergenic.

Rodents. Hamsters, guinea pigs, mice and rats are popular as pets and are also widely used in medical research. The major allergen occurs in their urine. Atopic subjects commonly become sensitized and react within a year of first exposure.

Horses and cows. Horse allergen is very potent, but most people can easily avoid horses. Cross-reactivity exists between horse dander and the serum used in tetanus vaccine.

Cow allergy is primarily a problem for people who work with cows (e.g. vets, farmers and cowboys). These individuals are, however, still able to eat beef.

Birds

'Feather allergy' is, in fact, mainly caused by exposure to mites that contaminate feathers. Allergy to bird droppings occurs in people who keep budgerigars or pigeons in poorly ventilated rooms. Bird antigens can cause allergic alveolitis. IgE-mediated allergy, resulting in asthma and rhinitis, is rarely a problem.

CHAPTER 3
Diagnosing allergy

History

Allergy diagnosis requires that a careful patient history is taken (Table 3.1), supported by investigations such as skin-prick tests.

Skin-prick testing

Skin-prick testing is an extremely useful test. When the allergen, introduced into the skin, interacts with IgE bound to mast cells, it causes histamine release and a consequent 'wheal-and-flare' (oedema and erythema) reaction (Figure 3.1).

Performance. A single drop of glycerinated extract is placed on the skin, which is punctured by a 1 mm lancet held at 90° to the skin surface. This test is simple, quick, virtually painless and has a high degree of specificity. Precision can be improved if the test is performed in duplicate.

Controls. A negative control with the diluent only is used to judge the extent of the reaction to the prick procedure itself. This may be large in patients with sensitive skin (dermographism). A positive control with histamine is used to judge skin reactivity and to discover whether there is any interfering antihistamine medication.

Allergen extract. It is advisable to use standardized extracts with consistent potency from a recognized supplier. The strength is usually given in biological units (BU) or in allergy units (AU) per ml.

Safety. Although skin-prick testing practically never causes problems, it is mandatory to have adrenaline available.

Influencing factors. Antihistamines depress skin reactivity and treatment must be stopped 4 days prior to testing. Topical corticosteroids on the skin

TABLE 3.1

Patient history for diagnosis of allergy

- Family history
  - eczema
  - asthma
  - rhinitis
  - urticaria
- Past history
  - eczema
  - asthma
  - rhinitis
  - urticaria
- Major nasal symptoms (sneezing, rhinorrhoea or blockage) and any other associated symptoms
- Timing
  - diurnal variation
  - seasonal variation
- Provoking and relieving factors
- Living conditions
  - house (age, dampness)
  - carpets, central heating
  - bedding, feathers
  - pets
- Occupation
  - exposure to allergen and irritants
  - relation of symptoms to work exposure
- Medication
  - present treatment
  - reactions to medication (e.g. aspirin)

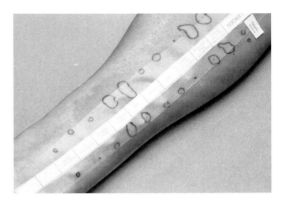

Figure 3.1 Skin-prick testing is the most important allergy examination. A positive test consists of a 'wheal-and-flare' reaction.

also reduce reactivity though systemic corticosteroids only do so in high doses (about 30 mg per day).

Reading the reaction (Figure 3.2). Maximum histamine reaction occurs at 10 minutes, and the allergen reaction occurs at 15 minutes. A reaction site with diameter 3 mm bigger than the negative control is usually taken to be positive. If a permanent record is required, the wheal can be outlined by felt-tip pen and the markings transferred to squared paper by means of tape.

Skin-prick testing must be interpreted in light of the patient's history. A positive skin-prick test can occur in a symptom-free subject (latent allergy), but this indicates an increased risk of later symptom development (10-fold in the case of grass pollen). For a symptomatic patient, exposure to allergen causing a positive skin-prick test will usually be of clinical significance. However, the skin test will remain positive after the cessation of symptoms and after immunotherapy.

Aero-allergen skin-prick test reactivity correlates well with symptoms. This is not the case for food allergens, where false-positive skin-prick test reactions often occur. The best way to diagnose food allergy is by dietary exclusion and re-introduction. Attempts to diagnose food allergy in a patient with symptoms of rhinitis will very rarely lead to clinical benefit.

Measurement of specific IgE antibody

The RAST (Radio Allergo Sorbent Test) was the first laboratory test for allergen-specific IgE in serum. The more recent version (Pharmacia's CAP System) has increased sensitivity.

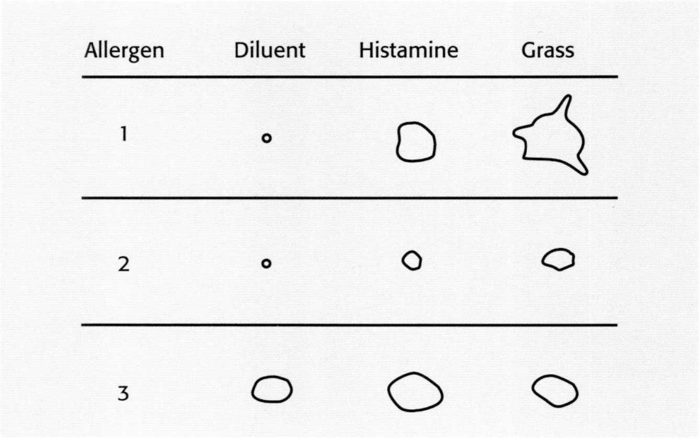

Figure 3.2 Reading the skin-prick test. Skin-prick testing for allergy to grass pollen. 1 = A clear positive test with the pollen reaction larger than the positive control with histamine; 2 = a false negative test with a very small reaction to histamine due to use of an oral antihistamine before testing; 3 = a false positive test in a patient reacting to the diluent due to dermographism.

The advantages of blood testing include absolute safety, standardization, a high degree of precision, independence from patient medication and lack of side-effects (such as causing increased itching in eczema patients). The disadvantages include high cost and lack of immediately available results. The measurement of specific IgE is no more sensitive than skin-prick testing. It can be used when skin-prick testing is unavailable or inadvisable, such as in patients taking antihistamines or with severe atopic dermatitis. It can also be used as a supplement to skin testing where there is doubt regarding the clinical significance of the result and when a confirmatory test is needed (e.g. prior to immunotherapy).

Allergen provocation test

This challenge test of nose or eye is useful for the study of pathophysiology and pharmacodynamics, but is rarely used diagnostically.

Total serum IgE

Normal values of IgE vary widely with age and there is a considerable overlap between atopic and non-atopic individuals. Most patients with

Nervous control

Adrenergic fibres in sympathetic nerves cause contraction of blood vessels when stimulated. Alpha-receptor agonists (sympathomimetics) are therefore used as nasal decongestants. Overuse of these can lead to reduced adrenergic responsiveness and rhinitis medicamentosa.

Parasympathetic nerves involve cholinergic fibres and stimulation of these causes hypersecretion from submucosal glands that can be inhibited by atropine and ipratropium bromide.

The nasal sensory nerves are constantly being stimulated by pollutants, temperature changes and atmospheric dryness, and there is a constant reflex activity that stimulates mucus production, modulates blood vessel tone and alters nasal patency. Thus a certain degree of nasal symptoms is a normal phenomenon. It can be difficult to make a clear distinction between a

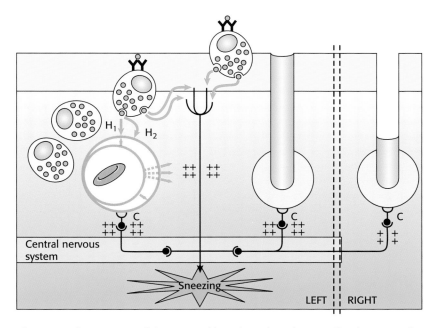

Figure 4.4 The response of the nose to histamine. Histamine acts directly on vascular receptors causing vasodilatation (H_1 and H_2 receptors), plasma exudation and oedema formation (H_1 receptors). Histamine stimulates sensory nerves (H_1 receptors) and initiates a parasympathetic reflex via cholinergic receptors (C), which results in hypersecretion in both sides of the nose.

normal physiological phenomenon and a rhinitis disease because individual acceptance of nasal symptoms varies considerably.

CHAPTER 5
Therapeutic principles

The treatment of rhinitis falls into four categories:
- allergen avoidance
- pharmacotherapy
- immunotherapy
- surgery (see pages 42 and 45).

Allergen avoidance

Although it is not practicable to avoid allergen exposure completely (Figure 5.1), the allergen load can usually be reduced. In principle, this is the first measure to take, particularly when the patient is a child. Allergen avoidance reduces the need for drug therapy and may reduce the risk of progression to asthma.

House-dust mite. Avoidance measures are needed particularly in the bedroom. Allergen-proof bedding reduces rhinitis and asthma symptoms by 50% and also has a beneficial effect on eczema (Table 5.1). Reducing a high indoor humidity, though difficult, can help to decrease the number of mites.

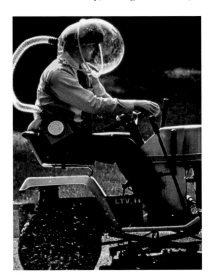

Figure 5.1 Although allergen avoidance, in principle, is the first step in allergic rhinitis therapy, it is not always feasible.

TABLE 5.1

House-dust mite avoidance in the bedroom

- Have linoleum or wooden flooring, which is smooth and easy to clean
- Only allow simple furniture and washable curtains
- Avoid all unnecessary dust-collecting items
- Replace old box spring mattresses with new ones
- Cover mattresses with allergen non-permeable covers
- Replace old feather pillows with new ones made from a synthetic material
- Cover pillows with allergen non-permeable covers or wash regularly
- Replace old quilts with new ones and wash regularly (> 55°C)
- Replace old eiderdowns with new ones and encase them
- Clean, vacuum and change bed linen regularly

Pets. Avoiding pets is easy – in principle at least. However, patients do not always follow their physician's advice.

Family pets should be kept out of bedrooms at all times, but this measure is not sufficient as most, particularly cats, are a source of potent allergens that are light and become distributed throughout the home. It may take months after the animal has been removed for the full benefit to be felt.

Indirect exposure from animal protein on other peoples' clothes, for example, in schools, cannot be avoided. This can cause problems in highly sensitive patients.

Pollens. These are more difficult to avoid but judicious use of holiday time can be helpful, as can closing windows and using car air filters.

Pharmacotherapy

The drugs available for use in rhinitis are:
- antihistamines
- corticosteroids
- cromoglycate

- vasoconstrictors
- cholinoceptor antagonists
- anti-leukotrienes.

Oral antihistamines. First-generation H_1-receptor antagonists were developed from tranquillizers and all caused some degree of sedation or psychomotor impairment. They have now been replaced largely by second-generation H_1 blockers, which are non-sedating or marginally sedating. These include loratadine, cetirizine, acrivastine, ebastine, fexofenadine and mizolastine (terfenadine and astemizole).

Pharmacology. These drugs are rapidly absorbed from the gastrointestinal tract and their onset of effect is within 1 hour (with the exception of astemizole). They are metabolized by the hepatic cytochrome P450 system. Cetirizine is an exception, being excreted unchanged in the urine. In addition, fexofenadine is only metabolized to a very low degree. Most drugs are effective in a single daily dose, giving good patient compliance (acrivastine needs to be given three times daily).

Clinical effects. Whilst effective against eye and nasal itching, sneezing and nasal running, these agents have little effect on nasal blockage. They are more effective in seasonal allergic rhinitis than in perennial disease, where blockage is a greater problem.

First-generation antihistamines cause sedation and can also cause significant psychomotor impairment without sedation. This can lead to serious errors when driving or operating machinery. Most individuals do not notice significant sedation with the second-generation drugs, though a minority still do.

Side-effects. Terfenadine and astemizole, if blood levels are raised, can cause prolongation of the QT interval and lead to serious ventricular tachycardia. This can occur in overdose situations or where metabolism is impaired by liver disease or by competing drugs such as ketoconazole, erythromycin or by grapefruit juice. It is also more likely if there are pre-existing cardiac problems or low potassium levels.

Topical antihistamines. The recent development of topical antihistamines for use in the eyes and nose has meant that quick relief of itching and sneezing can be obtained without risk of systemic side-effects. The major preparations currently available are levocabastine and azelastine, which can be given twice daily or on an as-needed basis.

Topical corticosteroids. Intranasal corticosteroids are the most effective medication presently available for the treatment of allergic rhinitis and some kinds of idiopathic rhinitis. Their major limitations are a relatively slow onset of action and the lack of effect on eye symptoms. Topical steroid treatment can be first-line therapy in moderate to severe hay fever, adult perennial allergic rhinitis and perennial idiopathic (non-allergic) rhinitis, and in nasal polyposis.

This treatment can be used once daily, giving a good patient compliance. There is a degree of systemic absorption from the nose, but systemic side-effects are not a problem at routine doses in adults. When steroids are used in children, it is important to use the lowest dosage that can control the symptoms and to give it once daily, in the morning. There do not seem to be any major differences between the modern corticosteroid molecules (e.g. beclomethasone diproprionate, flunisolide, budesonide, fluticasone proprionate, triamcinolone acetonide, mometasone furoate) in terms of efficacy and side-effects.

Betamethasone drops can be effective at the start of treatment or as part of a medical polypectomy. Their high systemic absorption and the tendency to overuse because of the lack of metering means that short-term use only is recommended. They should be avoided in children and pregnancy. Fluticasone proprionate, which is absorbed much less than betamethasone, recently has become available in drop formulation for use in nasal polyposis.

Side-effects. Initial sneezing and irritation may occur, largely due to nasal hyper-reactivity, but these should decrease with time. Dryness and bloodstained crusting in the anterior part of the nose occur in around 10% of patients, but can be reduced by proper use of the spray so that it does not impinge on the same point of the septum every time. If epistaxis occurs and is severe, stopping the spray for a few days, ointment in the nose and changing the formulation may help.

Twenty-five years of use have shown that there is no risk of atrophic rhinitis developing with long-term corticosteroid sprays but, rarely, a septal perforation can develop.

Children. Short-term use during the hay fever season is acceptable in childhood. In perennial allergic rhinitis, intranasal corticosteroids may be needed at the start of therapy or for those with severe disease. The lowest dose that can control the symptoms is given once daily, in the morning.

Pregnancy. No medication, including intranasal steroids, is considered 100% safe during pregnancy, particularly during the first trimester. Obviously the risk–benefit ratio for any prescription must be assessed but, in general, topical use is preferable to systemic agents and an established treatment is preferable to a new one.

Systemic corticosteroids. In severe cases, a short course of systemic corticosteroids can quickly reduce intranasal inflammation and lead to symptom relief, which can then be maintained with topical corticosteroids. Only short-term treatment (1–2 weeks) is used and courses should not be given more frequently than every 3–6 months. In principle, systemic corticosteroids are not used instead of other treatments, but in addition to a basic medication.

Prednisolone, 5–15 mg per day, can be given orally. Corticosteroids are also available as a depot injection (e.g. methylprednisolone, 40–80 mg). In rare cases, a depot injection can cause tissue atrophy at the injection site. Depot injections of steroid into swollen nasal turbinates or polyps have been reported to cause blindness in a few patients and must, therefore, be avoided.

The major areas of use of systemic corticosteroids are:
- at the start of treatment if nasal obstruction is severe
- in the pollen season when counts are very high
- as part of a medical polypectomy.

Contraindications include glaucoma, herpetic keratitis, diabetes mellitus, severe hypertension, advanced osteoporosis, psychic instability and active tuberculosis. Systemic steroids should not be used for rhinitis in children, or during pregnancy.

Cromoglycate/nedocromil sodium. These have weak activity in terms of symptom relief and require twice to four times daily dosing. They are both poorly absorbed and virtually free from side-effects. Cromoglycate is available as a nasal spray and as eye drops, nedocromil as eye drops. The major area of use is for perennial allergic rhinitis in children.

Topical vasoconstrictors/decongestants. Alpha-adrenoceptor agonists cause blood vessel constriction and therefore decongest the nose. They are best given intranasally.

Onset of action is quick and, in the cases of xylometazoline and oxymetazoline, prolonged (6–8 hours). However, patients like these sprays and tend to overuse them. These agents do have a place in treatment both at the start of treatment if the nose is very congested, and during the obstructive phase of colds and sinusitis. Regular, long-term use can result in rhinitis medicamentosa, in which there is rebound nasal congestion and hyper-reactivity. Use must, therefore, be restricted to 1 week.

Oral vasoconstrictors/decongestants. Although less effective than topical agents, the oral formulations are not associated with rhinitis medicamentosa.

Unfortunately the dose needed to treat a stuffy nose is at the borderline with that causing systemic side-effects, such as restlessness, difficulty in sleeping, tachycardia, palpitations and tremor. Oral vasoconstrictors are not suitable for patients with hypertension, coronary disease, prostatism, thyrotoxicosis, glaucoma and diabetes mellitus. They must not be used at the same time as monoamine oxidase inhibitors. Combined preparations of alpha-agonists (which can relieve nasal blockage) and antihistamines (which can relieve itching, sneezing and rhinorrhoea) are available.

Cholinoceptor antagonists. Isolated watery rhinorrhoea that is not associated with itch or sneezing rarely responds to the above therapies. However, as watery discharge is mediated via cholinergic receptors in the nasal glands, antagonists of these receptors are effective. Ipratropium bromide is available as a nasal spray. It is useful for watery rhinorrhoea in isolation and rhinorrhoea induced by hot, spicy food or exposure to cold air, and can be helpful in the common cold.

The dose needs to be adjusted for symptom severity and timing (most patients experience rhinorrhoea in the mornings). The major side-effect is nasal dryness, which can be alleviated by a saline spray.

Anti-leukotrienes. These drugs, which have just become available (montelukast and zafirlukast, in the UK, and zileuton and pranlukast, available only in the USA to date), are effective when taken orally for both asthma and rhinitis. They can be particularly helpful for the relief of nasal blockage and restoring the sense of smell. Their place in treatment is as yet uncertain, though they are likely to play a role in the treatment of aspirin-sensitive rhinitics with nasal polyps.

Nasal douching

Normally the nose cleans itself adequately using the mucociliary apparatus. However, mucociliary function is impaired during infection and in chronic rhinitis. Nasal douching, using an isotonic solution (one teaspoon of salt in 500 ml of water), is particularly beneficial in chronic infective rhinosinusitis. It can also alleviate nasal dryness.

Immunotherapy

Allergen-specific immunotherapy (allergen vaccination) comprises regular subcutaneous injections of allergen in a formulation designed to reduce allergic sensitization and consequently reduce symptoms in the nose, eyes and chest.

Indications. Immunotherapy is effective in patients suffering from pollen, animal and, to a lesser extent, mite allergy. It is as yet uncertain whether immunotherapy alters the natural history of allergic diseases and its place in therapy is controversial.

Before immunotherapy can be considered, the patient must be diagnosed with a skin-prick test or RAST and a history of symptom exacerbation on exposure to that particular allergen should be ascertained.

Young adults and children over 5 years of age are probably the best candidates for such treatment; in the elderly, the results are less impressive and side-effects more common.

Pollens. Controlled studies have shown efficacy with grass, birch, ragweed, mugwort, parietaria and cedar in the treatment of rhinoconjunctivitis and asthma.

Patients with severe rhinitic symptoms not controlled by pharmaco-therapy should be considered for immunotherapy, particularly if the allergen season is long.

Animal proteins. Avoidance is the major mode of treatment for these patients, but occasionally this is impossible (e.g. farmers, vets, laboratory workers or schoolchildren exposed to pet dander on the clothing of their classmates). Immunotherapy may be useful for these individuals, but it should not be a substitute for allergen avoidance.

House-dust mite. Controlled trials in adults have not shown definite efficacy with house-dust extracts, though studies in children have. Immunotherapy may be tried in young people who still have severe rhinitis symptoms despite mite avoidance measures and symptomatic therapy.

Contraindications. Patients with severe asthma or with a significant irreversible airways disease (FEV_1 < 70%) should not be given immunotherapy because of the risk of serious allergen-induced bronchoconstriction. The ideal patient is a young person with severe rhinitis and either no or mild asthma.

Good compliance is vital and those individuals who cannot attend regularly or who are alcohol or drug abusers should not be included on an immunotherapy programme. Other serious risk factors are the presence of cardiovascular disease and the use of beta-blockers.

Mechanism of action. A series of immunological changes associated with immunotherapy have been described, but it is uncertain which, if any of these, are related to efficacy.

Extracts. Only one or at most two allergens should be used, based on the results of allergy testing, knowledge of allergens in the patient's local environment and the potential for avoidance.

High-quality, standardized allergen extracts with little batch-to-batch variation should be used. Aqueous extracts require many injections and cause frequent systemic reactions. Depot extracts, in which aluminium hydroxide or tyrosine has been used to alter the nature of allergen, cause delayed absorption; fewer injections are required and the risk of systemic reaction is reduced.

Technique. Immunotherapy has two phases:
- increasing dose
- maintenance.

With depot preparations, the first phase comprises weekly injections, while maintenance injections are 6–8 weeks apart. During the increasing-dose phase, the dose is doubled with each injection when the preceding injection has caused little reaction. If there is a large local reaction or a systemic reaction, either the same dose is given again or a lower dose is given and the doses are increased more slowly. The optimal dose for maintenance injections is the highest dose tolerated without significant side-effects. This must be given at regular intervals and a strict safety regimen must be followed (see below).

With an aqueous extract, rush desensitization can be undertaken with the patient hospitalized receiving 2–6 injections daily over 1 week.

Pollen immunotherapy can either be given pre-seasonally, usually with weekly doses, or perennially, requiring few injections in the long term. The duration of treatment is usually 3–5 years.

Precautions. Every immunotherapy injection is associated with a risk of systemic allergic reaction, such as anaphylaxis or severe bronchospasm. Full cardiorespiratory resuscitation facilities must be to hand, together with adrenaline. The patient must be observed for at least 30 minutes following each injection (1 hour in the UK). Those with an asthma episode or those who are suffering from a cold or other systemic illness should not receive injections.

CHAPTER 6

Seasonal allergic rhinitis

Seasonal allergic rhinitis, also known as hay fever, is caused by allergy to pollen grains. In the northern hemisphere, tree pollens cause spring symptoms, grass pollen summer symptoms and in the early autumn weed pollens are the causative agent (see Figure 2.2). Pollen grains are mainly trapped in the nose and also land on the eye, so rhinoconjunctivitis is the major problem.

Occurrence

About 20% of the population are affected at some time during their lives. The disease usually starts in childhood or teenage years, and people are most commonly affected in early childhood. There is usually a decrease in symptomatology by middle age, and very few elderly people are affected.

Symptoms

Nasal itch, sneezing and watery rhinorrhoea with mild or moderate nasal blockage are the predominant symptoms. Itching of the eyes is also common. Some more severely affected individuals will develop asthma when the pollen count is high. Such patients frequently show bronchial hyper-reactivity even outside the pollen season.

Symptom severity in the eyes and nose correlates with the pollen count, which is highest in sunny, dry weather. During the hottest part of the day, the pollen rises to 500 m and can travel several miles at that altitude. Thus people in urban areas can be affected.

Diagnosis

This can usually be made from the patient's history, confirmed by skin-prick testing if needed.

Treatment

Allergen avoidance. Allergen exposure can be reduced by avoiding areas where there is likely to be a lot of pollen, such as grassland. Car windows should be kept closed and a filter installed on the air intake.

Planning of holiday timetables at the height of the pollen season can reduce symptoms. Pollen exposure leads to more inflammation in the nose, which leads to more symptoms on further exposure. Many patients do not understand this and a simple explanation is often helpful.

Pharmacotherapy. The goal of treatment is a normal life. Occasional antihistamines are all that are needed in mildly affected individuals.

More severely affected patients will need an intranasal corticosteroid. Regular use, particularly if started a week pre-seasonally, will control nasal symptoms in the majority of patients. A daily treatment used for 2–3 months is suitable for children and adults. If eyes are affected, antihistamine or cromoglycate/nedocromil eye drops (not corticosteroids) are indicated. Bathing the eyes with saline also relieves symptoms.

For severely affected patients, a short course of a systemic steroid may be added when breakthrough symptoms occur. This is best given in the form of tablets (e.g. prednisolone 10 mg/day), which can be taken as needed.

Immunotherapy can be considered for patients whose symptoms are not adequately controlled by pharmacotherapy.

CHAPTER 7
Perennial rhinitis: allergic and non-allergic

Perennial rhinitis can be allergic or non-allergic (idiopathic). Within the non-allergic group, a subgroup of patients have nasal eosinophilia (and respond well to topical corticosteroids); those without nasal eosinophilia have what is sometimes called 'vasomotor rhinitis'.

Occurrence

It is difficult to find an exact figure for the prevalence of this condition as there is a grey area between normality and rhinitis. Between 5 and 10% of the population are thought to be affected. Perennial allergic rhinitis usually starts in childhood, while the idiopathic form usually starts during adult life. The course is less favourable than that of seasonal allergic rhinitis and the disease often becomes chronic.

Aetiology

Mite allergy is the major cause of perennial allergic rhinitis; animal allergy, particularly that caused by cats and dogs, is another common cause. Pollen allergy can cause perennial symptoms in the tropics and sub-tropics. Occupational rhinitis can be due to bakers' flour; other forms of occupational rhinitis usually occur together with asthma. Allergy to foods very rarely a cause of isolated rhinitis. The causes of perennial non-allergic rhinitis are unknown, and the term 'idiopathic' rhinitis is therefore appropriate.

Symptomatic patients exhibit nasal hyper-reactivity, which means that they 'over-respond' to non-specific stimuli and irritants, such as cold air, pollution, alcohol and spicy foods.

Some pregnant women develop a hormonal rhinosinusitis, usually in the last trimester, when symptoms, mainly nasal stuffiness, increase with the increased oestrogen level. This is a self-limiting condition, disappearing quickly after delivery. Most patients will not require treatment; for those who do, an occasional topical decongestant at bedtime may help sleep.

Symptoms

Symptoms are similar to those associated with hay fever, but eye itching is less common and nasal blockage more prominent. Elderly men tend to have profuse rhinorrhoea.

It is helpful to assess the number of sneezes, nose blowings and symptom duration during the day as measures of severity.

Signs

The face of a child with perennial rhinitis has characteristic features, with an open mouth and a high-arched palate, sometimes accompanied by overbite and dental malocclusion; an allergic crease may be seen across the lower third of the nose (Figures 7.1 and 7.2). This is caused by frequent touching with the hand to alleviate itching ('the allergic salute'; Figure 7.3). Interior examination of the nose usually reveals swollen, pale mucosa and

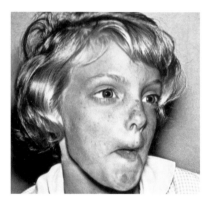

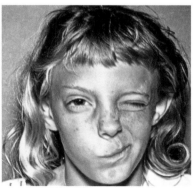

Figure 7.1 Mannerisms associated with the relief of nasal itching. Reproduced from Mark MB. *Stigmata of Respiratory Tract Allergens*. Kalamazoo: The Upjohn Company, 1972.

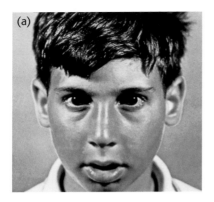
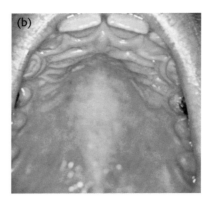

Figure 7.2 (a) 'Allergic shiners' and 'oedema bags' in a boy with perennial allergic rhinitis since infancy. (b) Chronic mouth breathing has resulted in an 'adenoidal face' and a high-arched palate. Reproduced from Mark MB. *Stigmata of Respiratory Tract Allergens*. Kalamazoo: The Upjohn Company, 1972.

clear fluid. The endoscope provides more information than the speculum and mirror.

Nasal patency can be estimated by rhinomanometry, acoustic rhinometry or nasal inspiratory peakflow, which provide accurate information used largely for research purposes.

Examinations

Skin-prick testing should be undertaken in all perennial rhinitis patients. A positive test that correlates with symptom exacerbation on allergen exposure leads to the correct allergy diagnosis.

Imaging. Sinus radiographs are no longer regarded as particularly helpful in the majority of rhinitis patients. The CT scan provides a much more precise tool for diagnosing anatomical abnormalities, nasal polyps and sinusitis, and for excluding differential diagnoses. It is not routinely indicated because of radiation exposure and cost. Most centres restrict its use to patients with chronic severe symptoms unresponsive to treatment, for excluding malignancy and in planning surgical intervention. It should be noted that a common cold may result in significant abnormalities in the nose and paranasal sinuses which may last for about 6 weeks.

(a)

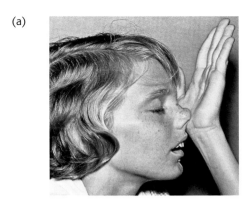

(b)

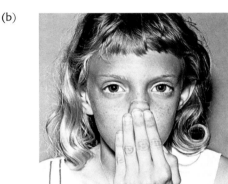

Figure 7.3 (a) The 'allergic salute' and (b) resulting 'nasal crease'. Reproduced from Mark MB. *Stigmata of Respiratory Tract Allergens*. Kalamazoo: The Upjohn Company, 1972.

Nasal cytology can be used to distinguish between eosinophilic and non-eosinophilic rhinitis, and between infectious and non-infectious rhinitis, although this test is rarely used in clinical practice. The most reproducible results are obtained with a disposable plastic curette (Rhinoprobe™) or a cytology brush. Both nostrils should be sampled. More than 10% eosinophils in the smear indicates nasal eosinophilia.

Therapy
Allergen avoidance is important, particularly in children in whom it might possibly prevent or delay progression to asthma.

Antihistamines. Oral and topical antihistamines are less useful in perennial than in seasonal rhinitis, but can be helpful when symptoms are intermittent such as on animal exposure.

Intranasal corticosteroids. Many patients with perennial allergic rhinitis show considerable improvement on a regular steroid spray. The same is true in patients with perennial idiopathic rhinitis. Not all of these patients will respond to topical corticosteroids – eosinophilia in nasal smears predicts a good result.

If blockage is pronounced at the start of treatment, a short course of oral steroids is indicated to open up the nose to permit access of the spray. Occasionally this can transform a non-responder to a responder.

Ipratropium nasal spray is useful in patients with predominant watery rhinorrhoea. One or two doses into each nostril should be given first thing in the morning, with additional doses spaced throughout the rest of the day as needed.

Saline douches can help patients with recurrent or chronic rhinosinusitis. Intranasal Vaseline helps when the vestibule is irritated by chronic rhinorrhoea; use of an antibacterial cream helps if there is infective (usually staphylococcal) vestibulitis.

Immunotherapy can be considered in children and youngsters not adequately controlled by allergen avoidance and pharmacotherapy. The ideal patient has severe rhinitis and mild asthma, not the reverse.

Surgery is rarely needed for patients with allergic rhinitis. However, when medical treatment has failed, turbinate reduction and/or attention to a deviated septum may prove helpful, particularly for allowing better access for nasal sprays. Endoscopic sinus surgery is now the treatment of choice for patients with chronic rhinosinusitis in whom ostiomeatal complex drainage has become compromised and who have not responded to several weeks of medical treatment.

CHAPTER 8
Nasal polyposis: a non-allergic disease

Nasal polyps are prolapsed, oedematous, mucous membranes that arise from the middle meatus, the area lateral to the middle turbinate. This region is close to the ostiomeatal complex (Figure 8.1). This is important for the normal function of the paranasal sinuses and the development of sinus pathology and sinusitis symptoms, which are often associated with polyposis.

Incidence
Approximately 1–2% of the population suffer from nasal polyposis with multiple polyps, which are part of a hyperplastic rhinosinusitis. However, careful endoscopic examination reveals small, isolated polyps in many individuals.

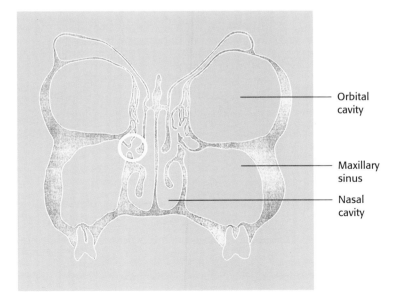

Orbital
cavity

Maxillary
sinus

Nasal
cavity

Figure 8.1 A front view of the ostiomeatal complex. This localized area, having the openings to the paranasal sinuses, is of utmost importance for sinus pathology. Its function is compromised by nasal polyps, formed in the middle meatus.

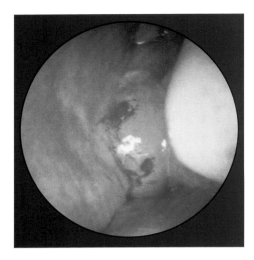

Figure 8.2 A nasal polyp seen at rhinoscopy (nasal endoscopy). It is pear-shaped with a stalk in the middle meatus and is pale yellow (plasma-filled sack) with a glistening surface. When touched by an instrument, it is soft, non-tender, and can be moved unlike the nasal mucous membrane.

Classification

Nasal polyps characteristically occur in patients with idiopathic rhinitis (with eosinophilia), non-allergic asthma and aspirin intolerance. A positive skin-prick test to aero-allergens is not more common in patients with nasal polyposis than in the background population and the term 'allergic polyps' is inaccurate, although histologically they are composed of eosinophilic inflammatory tissue.

Nasal polyposis is also a feature of chronic infective rhinitis. Patients with cystic fibrosis or primary ciliary dyskinesia often have polyps. Malignancy can present as nasal polyps.

Diagnosis

This is usually made by rhinoscopy (Figure 8.2). Polyps are bilateral and usually multiple. Histological examination is necessary at initial presentation of polyps in case there is underlying malignancy.

Polyps presenting in childhood should lead to a search for cystic fibrosis. An adult with nasal polyposis should be questioned about sensitivity to acetylsalicylic acid and other non-steroidal anti-inflammatory drugs.

CT scans

Prior to surgery, patients with nasal polyposis usually have a CT scan to both determine the extent of disease and look for any underlying factors,

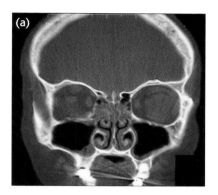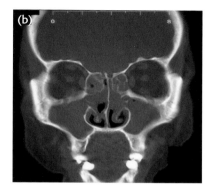

Figure 8.3 CT scans (a) in a patient with an early stage of nasal polyposis and (b) in a patient with an advanced stage.

such as malignancy and fungi, which chelate metals and cause areas of calcification in the polyp tissue (Figure 8.3).

Clinical presentation

Nasal obstruction is the major symptom, together with loss of smell. Rhinitic symptoms, such as running and sneezing, also occur, particularly in the early stage of the disease.

Characteristically, a patient will suffer from perennial non-allergic rhinitis for a number of years prior to the development of nasal polyposis; this can be complicated by the later development of intrinsic asthma.

Imaging shows that the sinus mucosa is thickened, hypertrophied and polypoid; sinus opacification is a usual finding (see Figure 8.3). Infective sinusitis can sometimes complicate this situation.

Treatment

Surgical. At initial presentation, surgery is needed to remove polyps for histological examination. Patients in whom some normal mucosa remains may well respond best to endoscopic surgery. Otherwise a simple snare polypectomy will suffice (Figure 8.4).

Isolated polyps (e.g. choanal and antrochoanal) need to be removed as completely as possible. In the case of antrochoanal polyps, the root must be removed from the maxillary sinus or polyps will recur.

(a)

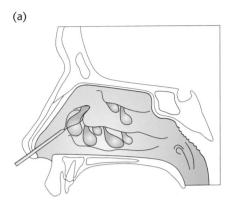

(b)

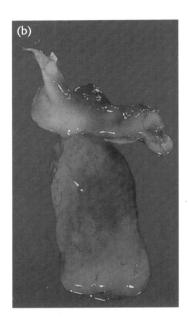

Figure 8.4 (a) A simple polypectomy using a snare. (b) A nasal polyp removed with a snare.

Medical. A short course of systemic corticosteroids, over 2 weeks, together with intranasal corticosteroids, can cause massive polyp shrinkage ('medical polypectomy') and dramatic symptom reduction. After this, long-term topical corticosteroids can prevent polyp recurrence.

Medical polypectomy is extremely effective on the first occasion, but should not be repeated within 3 months to avoid systemic side-effects.

After surgical intervention, patients should be put onto long-term topical corticosteroids. Many patients are maintained on medical treatment with the occasional need for surgical intervention. Unfortunately, local application of steroids, in contrast to systemic administration, has little or no effect on the sense of smell. This side-effect, which often also manifests as a loss of taste, is very irritating to the patient. Recently, recovery of olfaction has been noted in patients taking leukotriene-receptor antagonists in addition to corticosteroids (GS, personal observation).

CHAPTER 9
Associated diseases

Rhinitis is frequently disregarded and trivialized by physicians. However, quality-of-life studies show that it impairs quality of life more than mild to moderate asthma. As the epithelium of the nose continues down into the lungs, around the sinuses and up into the ears, it is not surprising that nasal disease can have secondary effects on these organs.

Asthma

Approximately 75% of asthmatics have rhinitis; conversely, 25% of patients with rhinitis have asthma. In a recent study, 50% of those with both diseases developed rhinitis first, with a mean gap of 2 years before the development of asthma. This points to possible asthma prevention.

Treatment of rhinitis in asthmatics with topical corticosteroids is associated with an improvement in asthma symptoms and a decrease in bronchial hyper-reactivity. Some patients with severe intractable asthma are found to have an underlying chronic sinusitis that, when treated, can make the asthma more manageable.

The underlying mechanism(s) linking these two diseases is not fully understood. Possibilities include:

- the loss of the air purification and warming mechanisms of the nose when mouth breathing supervenes
- postnasal dripping of inflammatory mediators during deep sleep
- release of cytokines and mediators from the nasal mucosa to the circulation
- 'homing' of inflammatory cells from the bone marrow in both the upper and lower airways
- a naso-sino-bronchial reflex.

That nitric oxide (NO) acts as an inflammatory mediator raises the possibility of its involvement between the nose and lungs, particularly as the NO concentration in the sinuses is several times higher than in the lungs.

Whatever the mechanism(s), it is advisable that rhinitis should be searched for in patients with asthma and, if present, treated effectively.

Sinusitis

'Rhinitis' is a shortened version of 'rhinosinusitis'; when nasal inflammation exists, the sinus mucosa is usually involved, to some extent, in the inflammatory process. In some patients, bacterial superinfection occurs. This may be secondary to blockage of the ostiomeatal complex at the level of the middle turbinate meatus into which the sinuses drain.

Otitis media with effusion

A proportion of children with recurrent otitis media with effusion have rhinitis, often allergic in character. A few studies have now shown that treatment of their noses with topical corticosteroids aids resolution of otitis media with effusion, probably because Eustachian tube function and middle ear ventilation are improved.

Pharyngitis/laryngitis

Patients who chronically breathe through their mouths have dry mouths and tend to suffer from sore throats. Postnasal secretions dripping down into the pharynx and on to the larynx can also cause irritation, resulting in coughing and hawking. This, in turn, results in further local irritation of the mucous membranes and thus a vicious circle is created. Such symptoms are very difficult to resolve completely; postnasal passage of mucus is a normal phenomenon and once it has been noticed, the perception of it tends to persist even if the volume and stickiness of the secretions has been reduced by treatment of the rhinosinusitis.

Key references

GENERAL

Durham SR. *ABC of Allergies*. London: BMJ Publishing Group, 1998:1–66.

Holgate ST, Church MK. *Allergy*. London: Gower Medical Publishing, 1993.

Lund VJ, Aaronson D, Bousquet J *et al*. International consensus report on the diagnosis and management of rhinitis. *Allergy* 1992;49(suppl 19):1–34.

Mygind N, Dahl R, Pedersen S, Thestrup-Pedersen K. *Essential Allergy*. 2nd edn. Oxford: Blackwell Science, 1996.

Naclerio RM, Durham SR, Mygind N, eds. *Rhinitis. Mechanisms and Management*. New York: Marcel Dekker, 1999.

Scadding GK, Drakelee A, Durham SR *et al. Rhinitis. Management Guidelines*. 2nd edn. British Society for Allergy and Clinical Immunology, 1998.

ALLERGY: AN INCREASING PROBLEM

Arshad SH, Matthews S, Gant C *et al*. Effect of allergen avoidance on development of allergic disorders in infancy. *Lancet* 1992;339:1493–7.

Bentley AM, Jacobson MR, Cumberworth V *et al*. Immunohistology of the nasal mucosa in seasonal allergic rhinitis: increases in activated eosinophils and epithelial mast cells. *J Allergy Clin Immunol* 1992;89:877–83.

Björkstén B. Risk factors in early childhood for the development of atopic diseases. *Allergy* 1994;49:400–7.

Bousquet J, Burney P. Evidence for an increase in atopic disease and possible causes. *Clin Exp Allergy* 1993;23:484–92.

Busse WW, Holgate ST, eds. *Asthma and Rhinitis*. Oxford: Blackwell Scientific Publications, 1995.

Canonica GW, Buscaglia S, Pesce G *et al*. Adhesion molecules in allergic inflammation: recent insights into their functional role. *Allergy* 1994;49:135–41.

Del Prete G. Human Th1 and Th2 lymphocytes: their role in the pathophysiology of atopy. *Allergy* 1992;47:450–5.

Durham SR. Allergic inflammation. *Pediatr Allergy Immunol* 1993;4(suppl 4):7–12.

Frew AJ, O'Hehir R. What can we learn from studies of lymphocytes present in allergic sites? *J Allergy Clin Immunol* 1992;89:783–8.

Holgate ST, Church MK. The mast cells. *Br Med Bull* 1992;48:40–50.

Romagnani S. Induction of Th1 and Th2 responses: a key role for the natural immune response? *Immunology Today* 1992;13:379–81.

von Mutius E, Fritzsch C, Weiland SK *et al*. Prevalence of asthma and allergic disorders among children in united Germany: a descriptive comparison. *BMJ* 1992;305:1395–9.

Wickman M, Nordvall SL, Pershagen G. Risk factors in early childhood for sensitization to airborne allergens. *Pediatr Allergy Immunol* 1992;3:128–33.

ALLERGENS: THE CAUSES OF ALLERGY

D'Amato G, Spieksma FTM, Bonini S, eds. *Allergenic Pollen and Pollinosis in Europe*. Oxford: Blackwell Scientific Publications, 1991.

Del Prete GF, De Carli M, Délios MM *et al.* Allergen exposure induces activation of allergen-specific Th2 cells in the airway mucosa of patients with allergic respiratory disorders. *Eur J Immunol* 1993;23:1445–9.

DIAGNOSIS OF ALLERGY

Anonymous. From the Board of Directors. American Academy of Allergy and Clinical Immunology. Allergen skin testing. *J Allergy Clin Immunol* 1993;92:636–7.

Dreborg S, Frew A. Position paper: allergen standardization and skin tests. *Allergy* 1993;48(suppl 14):49–82.

PATHOGENESIS OF RHINITIS

Borres MP. Metachromatic cells and eosinophils in atopic children. A prospective study. *Pediatr Allergy Immunol* 1991;2(suppl 2):6–24.

Howarth PH, Wilson S, Lau L *et al.* The nasal mast cell and rhinitis. *Clin Exp Allergy* 1991;21(suppl 2):3–8.

Naclerio RM, Togias AG. The nasal allergic reaction: observations on the role of histamine. *Clin Exp Allergy* 1990;21(suppl 2):13–19.

Terada N, Konno A, Togawa K. Biochemical properties of eosinophils and their preferential accumulation mechanism in nasal allergy. *J Allergy Clin Immunol* 1994;94:629–42.

van Wijk RG. Nasal hyperreactivity: its pathogenesis and clinical significance. *Clin Exp Allergy* 1991;21:661–7.

Varney VA, Jacobson MR, Sudderick RM *et al.* Immunohistology of the nasal mucosa following allergen-induced rhinitis. *Am Rev Respir Dis* 1992;146:170–6.

THERAPEUTIC PRINCIPLES, SEASONAL ALLERGIC AND PERENNIAL RHINITIS

Bousquet J, Lockey R, Malling H-J. Allergen immunotherapy: Therapeutic vaccines for allergic diseases. A WHO position paper. *J Allergy Clin Immunol* 1998;102:558–62.

Church M. The therapeutic index of antihistamines. *Pediatr Allergy Immunol* 1993;4(suppl 4):25–32.

Coleman JW, Davies RJ, Durham SR *et al.* Position paper on allergen immunotherapy. Report of a BSACI working party. *Clin Exp Allergy* 1993;23(suppl 1):1–44.

Dechant KL, Goa KL. Levacabastine. *Drugs* 1991;41:202–24.

Durham SR, Varney V, Gaga M *et al.* Immunotherapy and allergic inflammation. *Clin Exp Allergy* 1991;21(suppl 1):206–10.

Dreborg S, Frew A. Position paper: allergen standardization and skin tests. *Allergy* 1993;48(suppl 14):49–54.

From the Food and Drug Administration. Warnings issued on nonsedating antihistamines terfenadine and astemizole. *JAMA* 1992;268:705.

Laursen LC, Faurschou P, Pals H *et al*. Intramuscular betamethasone dipropionate vs. oral prednisolone in hay fever patients. *Allergy* 1987;42:168–72.

Lund VJ. International consensus report on the diagnosis and management of rhinitis. *Allergy* 1994;49(suppl 19):1–34.

McTavich D, Sorkin EM. Azalastine: a review of its pharmacodynamic and pharmacokinetic properties, and therapeutic potential. *Drugs* 1989;38:778–88.

Meltzer E. The pharmacological basis for the treatment of perennial allergic rhinitis and non-allergic rhinitis with topical corticosteroids. *Allergy* 1997;52(suppl 36):33–40.

Mygind N, Lund V. Topical corticosteroid therapy of rhinitis: a review. *Clin Immunother* 1996;122:36.

Reid MJ, Lockey RF, Turkeltaub PC *et al*. Survey of fatalities from skin testing and immunotherapy 1985–1989. *J Allergy Clin Immunol* 1993;92:6–15.

Simons FER. The therapeutic index of newer H_2-receptor antagonists. *Clin Exp Allergy* 1994;24:707–23.

Taccariello M, Parikh A, Darby Y *et al*. Nasal douching as a valuable adjunct in the management of chronic rhinosinusitis. *Rhinology* 1999;37:29–32.

Varney VA, Gaga M, Frew AJ *et al*. Usefulness of immunotherapy in patients with severe summer hay fever uncontrolled by antiallergic drugs. *BMJ* 1991;302:265–9.

Weeks J, Oliver J, Birmingham K *et al*. A combined approach to reduce mite allergen in the bedroom. *Clin Exp Allergy* 1995;25:1179–83.

NASAL POLYPOSIS: A NON-ALLERGIC DISEASE

Mygind N, Lildholdt T, eds. *Nasal Polyposis. An Inflammatory Disease and its Treatment*. Copenhagen: Munksgaard, 1997:1–183.

Tos M, Svendstrup F, Arndal H *et al*. Efficacy of aqueous and a powder formulation of nasal budesonide compared in patients with nasal polyps. *Am J Rhinol* 1998;12:183–9.

ASSOCIATED DISEASES

Mygind N, Dahl R, eds. The nose and paranasal sinuses in asthma. *Allergy* 1999;54(suppl):1–235.

Rachelevsky GS, Katz RM, Siegel SC. Chronic sinus disease with associated reactive airway disease in children. *Pediatrics* 1984;73:526–9.

Townley RG, Kiboneka A. Allergic rhinitis: relationship to asthma: similarities, differences and interactions. *Ann Allergy Asthma Immunol* 1998;80:137–9.

Index

allergy 5
  causes 11–16
    see also allergens by name
  diagnosis 17–21
    patient history 18, 36
  increasing problem 7–10
  pathogenesis 22–6
  see also epidemiology; genetic
    factors; treatment
animals as allergens 9, 11, 15,
  28, 34, 38, 41
antihistamines 28, 29–30, 37,
  41
aspergillosis 21
aspirin intolerance 10, 44
asthma 5, 7, 8, 10, 21, 36, 42,
  44, 45, 47
atopic eczema 5, 7, 8, 21

birds as allergens 16
blood eosinophil count 21

childhood asthma 9
cockroaches 9, 15
corticosteroids 28, 30–1, 37, 38,
  42, 46, 47, 48
  contraindications 31
CT imaging 40, 44, 45
cytology 41

dermatitis see atopic eczema
dermatology 5
diesel exhaust 9, 10
drug allergy 21

environmental exposure 8–10
epidemiology 7–8
eye drops 31, 37

food allergy 19, 38

gases 9, 10, 23
genetic factors 8

hay fever see rhinitis, allergic,
  seasonal

histamine 24, 25
  see also antihistamines
house-dust mites 8, 9, 11,
  13–14, 27–8, 34, 38

IgE see immune reactions
immune reactions 7, 11, 19–20,
  23–4
inflammation, nasal 23–4, 48

lung medicine 5

moulds 9, 11, 13, 23

nasal eosinophilia 38, 41, 42, 44
  see also blood eosinophil
    count
nasal polyps 10, 21, 43–6
  classification 44
  clinical presentation 45
  CT scans 44–5
  diagnosis 44
  incidence 43
  treatment 30, 31, 45–6
nasal sprays 31, 32, 42

otitis media 48
otorhinolaryngology 5

pharyngitis/laryngitis 48
pollen 7, 11–13, 19, 23, 28, 31,
  33, 35, 36–7, 38
polypectomy 30, 31, 45–6

rhinitis, allergic 5, 7–10, 21, 29,
  30
  childhood 9, 10, 36, 38
  perennial 14, 31, 38–42
    aetiology 38
    examinations 40–1
    occurrence 38
    signs and symptoms 39–40
    therapy 41–2
  seasonal 7, 8, 12, 38, 41
    diagnosis 36
    occurrence 36

    symptoms 36–7
    treatment 36
rhinitis, chronic 24, 29
rhinitis, immediate 24
rhinitis, non-allergic 21, 38, 45
rhinitis, occupational 38
rhinoconjunctivitis 36
rhinorrhoea 32, 36, 39, 42
rhinosinusitis 33, 38, 40, 42, 43,
  47, 48

skin-prick test 7, 10, 17–19, 20,
  33, 36, 40
smoking, parental 9

treatment 27–35
  allergen avoidance 27–8, 34,
    36, 41
  immunotherapy 33–5, 37, 42
    contraindications 34
    precautions 35
  pharmacotherapy 28–33, 37
  surgery 42, 45

vasoconstrictors 32
  contraindications 32

Other titles available in the *Fast Facts* series

Asthma
by Stephen T Holgate and Romain A Pauwels

Allergic Rhinitis
by Niels Mygind and Glenis K Scadding

Benign Prostatic Hyperplasia (third edition)
by Roger S Kirby and John D McConnell

Coeliac Disease
by Geoffrey Holmes and Carlo Catassi

Contraception
by Anna Glasier and Beverly Winikoff

Diseases of the Testis
*by Timothy J Christmas, Michael D Dinneen and
Larry Lipshultz*

Dyspepsia
by Michael J Lancaster Smith and Kenneth L Koch

Endometriosis
by Hossam Abdalla and Botros Rizk

Epilepsy
by Martin J Brodie and Steven C Schachter

Headaches
by Richard Peatfield and J Keith Campbell

Hyperlipidaemia
by Paul Durrington and Allan Sniderman

Irritable Bowel Syndrome
by Kenneth W Heaton and W Grant Thompson

Menopause
by David H Barlow and Barry G Wren

Stress and Strain
by Cary L Cooper and James Campbell Quick

Urinary Continence
by Julian Shah and Gary Leach

To order, please contact:

Health Press Limited
Elizabeth House, Queen Street,
Abingdon, Oxford OX14 3JR, UK
Tel: +44 (0)1235 523233
Fax: +44 (0)1235 523238
Email: post@healthpress.co.uk

Or visit our website:
www.healthpress.co.uk

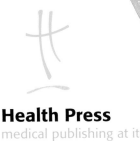

Health Press
medical publishing at its best

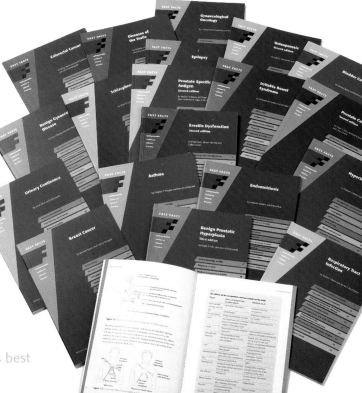